The Best Keto Slow Cooker Dessert Cookbook

A cookbook of dessert recipes for your keto slow cooker diet, to stay healthy

Lilith Wolfe

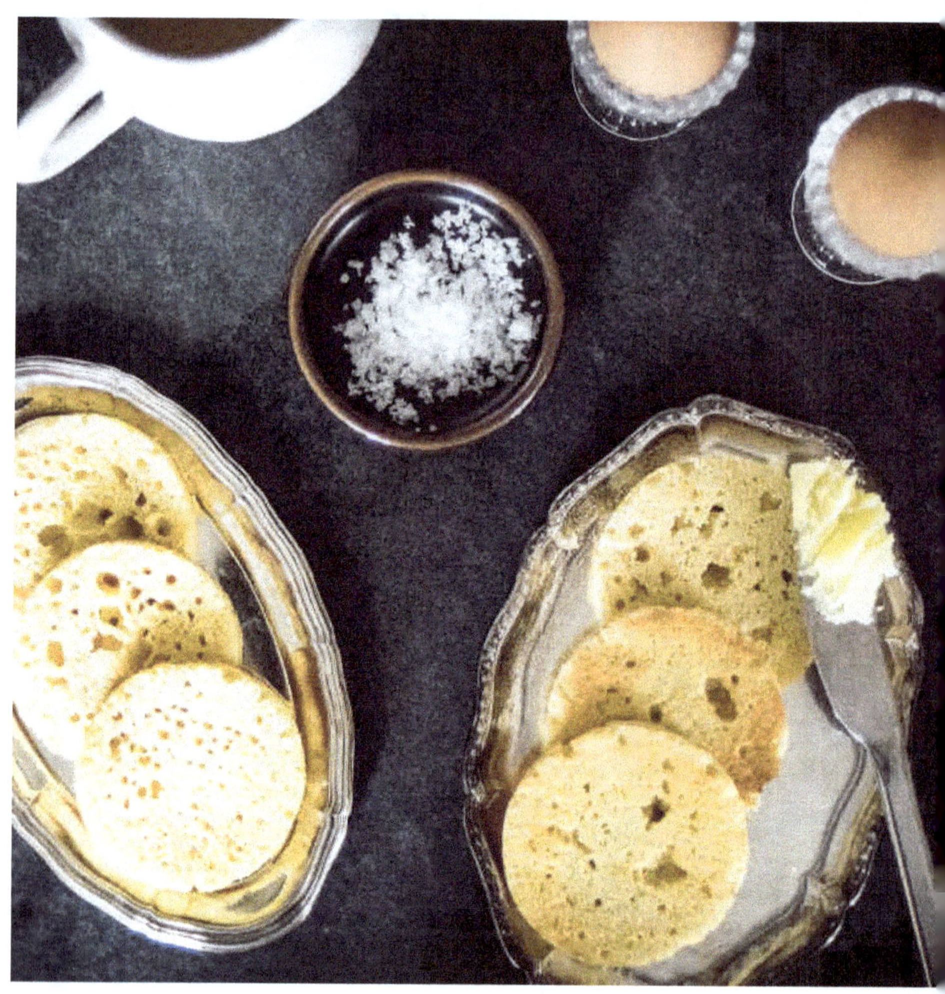

COPYRIGHT

indirectly. Respective authors own all copyrights not held by the publisher.

The information herein is offered for informational purposes solely and is universal as so. The presentation of the information is without contract or any type of guarantee assurance.

Table of contents

Tasty Apple and Cranberry Dessert

Preparation time: 15 minutes

Cooking time: 3 hours

Servings: 4

Ingredients:

4 medium-sized sliced apples

1 cup of frozen or fresh cranberries

1 teaspoon of vanilla

8 tablespoons of light brown packed sugar

2 teaspoons of ground cinnamon, divided

1 packet of super moist yellow cake mix, 15 ounces

8 tablespoons of melted butter

Whipped cream

Directions:

Grease the slow cooker. Add 1 teaspoon of cinnamon, brown sugar, apples, and cranberries to the slow cooker and combine them.

Mix the rest of 1 teaspoon of cinnamon with the dry cake mix in a bowl.

Spread the mixture onto the fruits and drizzle the melted butter over the top. Cook within 3 hours, on high. Serve it with whipped cream.

Nutrition:

Calories: 230 Fat: 12 gProtein: 30 g

Carbohydrates: 4.5 g

Caramel Pecan Pudding

Preparation time: 15 minutes

Cooking time: 3 hours

Servings: 4

Ingredients:

1 ½ cups of Bisquick mix

16 tablespoons of sugar, divided

8 tablespoons of unsweetened baking cocoa

8 tablespoons of milk

12 tablespoons of caramel topping, divided

1 2/3 cups of hot water

½ cup of chopped pecans

Directions:

Mix the Bisquick mix, 8 tablespoons of sugar, cocoa, milk, and 6 tablespoons of caramel in a large bowl.

Pour the mixture into a slow cooker. Add the hot water.

Top with the remaining sugar then cooks on low within 3 hours.

Divide into bowls, spread the remaining caramel over the top, sprinkle with pecans, and serve.

Nutrition:

Carbohydrates: 19 g Calories: 544

Fat: 5.6 g Protein: 3.4 g

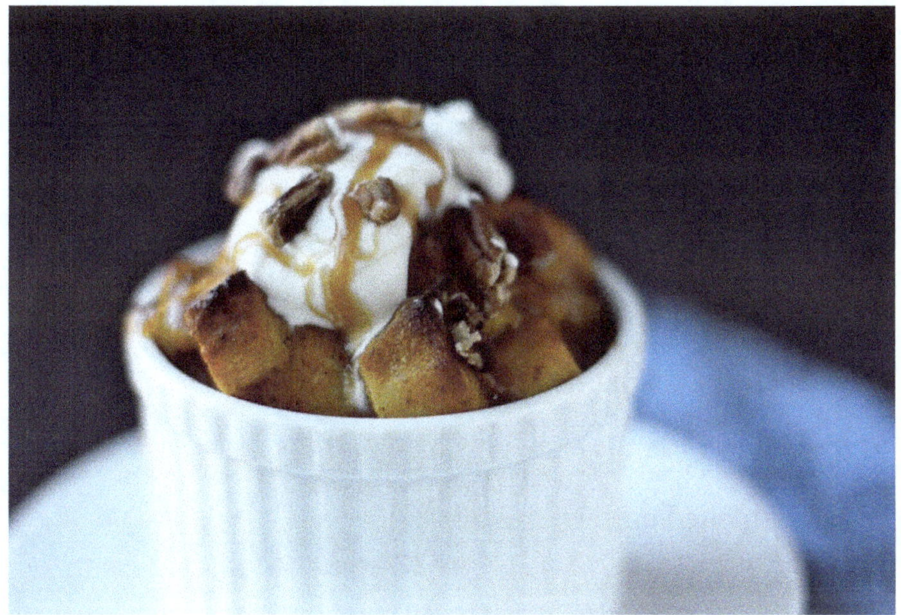

Mouth-Watering Chocolate Cake

Preparation time: 15 minutes

Cooking time: 3.5 hours

Servings: 4

Ingredients:

1 ½ cups of almond flour

¾ cup of granulated sugar or a sweetener of your preference

2/3 cup of cocoa powder

¼ cup of whey protein powder

2 teaspoons of baking powder

¼ teaspoons of salt

½ cup of melted butter

4 large eggs

¾ cup of unsweetened almond milk

1 teaspoon of vanilla extract

Whipped cream

Directions:

Mix the dry fixing in a large bowl.

Put the wet fixing to it one at a time, stirring as you go along. Whisk together thoroughly.

Grease the slow cooker and add the cake mixture—cover and cook for 3.5 hours on low.

Divide into bowls and serve with whipped cream.

Nutrition:

Calories: 260 Fat: 14 g

Protein: 8 g Carbohydrates: 15 g

Fabulous Peanut Vanilla Chocolate Butter Cake

Preparation time: 15 minutes

Cooking time: 4 hours

Servings: 4

Ingredients:

3/4 cup of melted natural peanut butter

4 large eggs

2 cups of almond flour

½ a cup of water

¼ cup of unflavored whey protein powder

½ cup of melted butter

2 ounces of melted dark chocolate, sugar-free

¾ cup of your preferred sweetener

¼ cup of coconut flour

1 teaspoon of vanilla extract

1 tablespoon of baking powder

¼ teaspoon of salt

1 teaspoon of vanilla extract

Directions:

Deglaze the inside of the slow cooker using a butter .

Combine all the **Ingredients** in a large bowl and whisk together thoroughly.

Spoon 2/3 of the batter onto the base of the slow cooker. Add half of the melted chocolate.

Add the remainder of the batter. Put the remaining chocolate on top.

Cover and cook for 4 hours. Divide onto plates and serve.

Nutrition:

Calories: 335

Carbohydrates: 11.5 g

Fat: 27 g

Fiber: 5.2 g

Protein: 8 g

Poppy Seed Butter Cake

Preparation time: 15 minutes

Cooking time: 3 hours

Servings: 4

Ingredients:

4 large eggs

The zest and juice of 4 lemons

½ cup of melted butter

2 cups of almond flour

3 tablespoons of poppy seeds

2 tablespoons of baking powder

1 tablespoon of vanilla extract

1 teaspoon of salt

½ cup of vanilla protein powder

3 tablespoons of vanilla protein powder

½ cup of xylitol

Directions:

Mix all the items except the eggs in a bowl.

Add the eggs one by one and whisk together thoroughly.

Grease the slow cooker with butter. Pour the batter into the slow cooker.

Cover and cook for 3 hours. Divide onto plates and serve.

Nutrition:

Calories: 143 Carbohydrates: 9 g

Fat: 10 g Fiber: 1 g

Protein: 6 g

Wonderful Raspberry Almond Cake

Preparation time: 15 minutes

Cooking time: 3 hours

Servings: 4

Ingredients:

1 cup of fresh raspberries

1/3 cup of dark chocolate chips, sugar-free

2 cups of almond flour

1 teaspoon of coconut extract

¾ cup of almond milk

4 large eggs

2 teaspoons of baking soda

¼ teaspoon of salt

1 cup of Swerve

½ cup of melted coconut oil

1 cup of shredded coconut unsweetened

¼ cup of powdered egg whites

Directions:

Grease the slow cooker with butter. Mix all the fixing in a bowl.

Pour the batter inside, then cook within 3 hours on low.

Nutrition:

Calories: 362

Carbohydrates: 12.8 g

Fat: 26 g

Protein: 8 g

Scrumptious Chocolate Cocoa Cake

Preparation time: 15 minutes

Cooking time: 4 hours

Servings: 4

Ingredients:

1 ½ cups of ground almonds

½ cup of coconut flakes

6 tablespoons of your preferred sweetener

2 teaspoons of baking powder

A pinch of salt

½ cup of coconut oil

½ cup of cooking cream

2 tablespoons of lemon juice

The zest from 2 lemons

2 large eggs

Espresso and whipped cream for serving

Toppings:

3 tablespoons of sweetener

½ a cup of boiling water

2 tablespoons of lemon juice

2 tablespoons of coconut oil

Directions:

Combine the baking powder, sweetener, coconut, and almonds in a large bowl. Whisk together thoroughly.

In another bowl, combine the eggs, juice, coconut oil, and whisk together thoroughly.

Combine the wet and the dry **Ingredients** and whisk together thoroughly.

Put the aluminum foil inside the bottom of the slow cooker. Pour the batter into the slow cooker.

Mix all the topping fixing in a small bowl, and pour on top of the cake batter.

Cover the slow cooker with paper towels to absorb condensation, then cook within 3 hours on high.

Divide into bowls and serve with espresso and whipped cream.

Nutrition:

Carbs: 5 g Protein: 7 g

Fat: 24 g

Lemon Cake

Preparation time: 15 minutes

Cooking time: 3 hours

Servings: 8

Ingredients:

1 ½ cup ground almonds

½ cup coconut flake s

6 Tablespoons sweetener like Swerve (Erythritol, or a suitable substitute)

2 teaspoons baking powder

Pinch of salt

½ cup softened coconut oil

½ cup cooking cream

2 Tablespoons lemon juice

Zest from two lemons

2 eggs

Topping:

3 tablespoons Swerve (or a suitable substitute)

½ cup boiling water

2 Tablespoons lemon juice

2 Tablespoons softened coconut oil

Directions:

In a bowl, combine the almonds, coconut, sweetener, baking powder. Whisk until combined.

In a separate bowl, blend coconut oil, cream, juice, and eggs.

Add the egg mixture to the dry fixing, mix.

Line the crockpot with aluminum foil, pour in the batter.

In a bowl, mix the topping. Pour it over the cake batter.

Cover it with paper towels to absorb the water.

Cover, cook on high for 3 hours. Serve warm.

Nutrition:

Calories: 142

Carbs: 0g

Fat: 8g

Protein: 0g

Raspberry & Coconut Cake

Preparation time: 15 minutes

Cooking time: 3 hours

Servings: 10

Ingredients:

2 cups ground almonds

1 cup shredded coconut

¾ cup sweetener, Swerve (or a suitable substitute)

2 teaspoon baking soda

¼ teaspoon salt

4 large eggs

½ cup melted coconut oil

¾ cup of coconut milk

1 cup raspberries, fresh or frozen

½ cup sugarless dark chocolate chips

Directions:

Butter the crockpot.

In a bowl, mix the dry **Ingredients**.

Beat in the eggs, melted coconut oil, and coconut milk. Mix in the raspberries plus chocolate chips.

Combine the cocoa, almonds, and salt in a bowl.

Pour the batter into the buttered crockpot.

Cover the crockpot with a paper towel to absorb the water.

Cover, cook on low for 3 hours. Let the cake cool in the pot.

Nutrition:

Calories: 201

Carbs: 24g Fat: 10g

Protein: 0g

Chocolate Cheesecake

Preparation time: 15 minutes

Cooking time: 2.5 hours

Servings: 8

Ingredients:

3 cups cream cheese

Pinch of salt

3 eggs

1 cup powder sweetener of your choice, Swerve (or a suitable substitute)

1 teaspoon vanilla extract

½ cup sugarless dark chocolate chips

Directions:

Whisk the cream cheese, sweetener, and salt in a bowl.

Add the eggs one at a time. Combine thoroughly.

Spread the cheesecake in a cake pan, which fits in the crockpot you are using.

Dissolved the chocolate chips in a small pot and pour over the batter. Using a knife, swirl the chocolate through the batter.

Put 2 cups of water inside the crockpot and set the cake pan inside. Cover it with a paper towel to absorb the water, then cook on high for 2.5 hours. Remove from the crockpot and let it cool in the pan for 1 hour. Refrigerate.

Nutrition:

Calories: 330 Carbs: 34g

Fat: 19g

Protein: 6g

Crème Brule

Preparation time: 15 minutes

Cooking time: 2 hours

Servings: 6

Ingredients:

5 large egg yolks

6 Tablespoons sweetener, Erythritol

2 cups double cream

1 Bourbon vanilla pod, scraped

Pinch of salt

Directions:

In a bowl, beat the eggs and sweetener together.

Add the cream and vanilla. Whisk together.

Put it in one big dish.

Set it in the crockpot and pour hot water around- so the water reaches halfway up the dish.

Cover, cook on high for 2 hours.

Take the dishes out, let them cool. Refrigerate for 6-8 hours.

Nutrition:

Calories: 120

Carbs: 18g

Fat: 4g

Protein: 3g

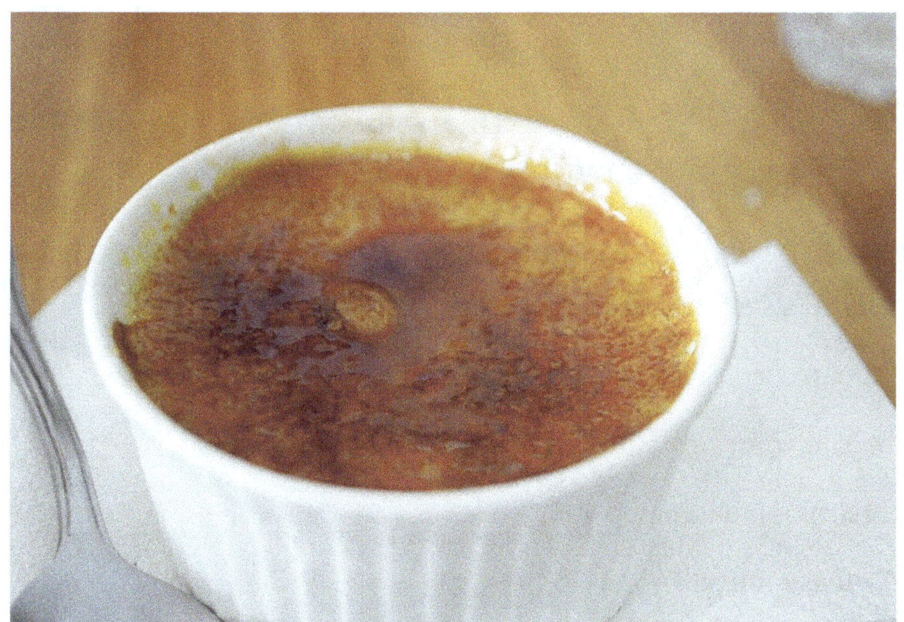

Peanut Butter & Chocolate Cake

Preparation time: 15 minutes

Cooking time: 4 hours

Servings: 12

Ingredients :

1 Tablespoon butter for greasing the crockpot

2 cups almond flour

¾ cup sweetener of your choice

¼ cup coconut flakes

¼ cup whey protein powder

1 teaspoon baking powder

¼ teaspoon salt

¾ cup peanut butter, melted

4 large eggs

1 teaspoon vanilla extract

½ cup of water

3 Tablespoons sugarless dark chocolate, melted

Directions:

Grease the crockpot well.

In a bowl, mix the dry **Ingredients**. Stir in the wet **Ingredients** one at a time.

Spread about 2/3 of batter in the crockpot, add half the chocolate. Swirl with a fork. Top up with the remaining batter and chocolate. Swirl again.

Cook on low for 4 hours. Switch off. Let it sit covered for 30 minutes.

Nutrition:

Calories: 270

Carbs: 39g

Fat: 11g

Protein: 5g

Berry & Coconut Cake

Preparation time: 15 minutes

Cooking time: 2 hours

Servings: 8

Ingredients:

1 Tablespoon butter for greasing the crock

1 cup almond flour

¾ cup sweetener of your choice

1 teaspoon baking soda

¼ teaspoon salt

1 large egg, beaten with a fork

¼ cup coconut flour

¼ cup of coconut milk

2 Tablespoons coconut oil

4 cups fresh or frozen blueberries and raspberries

Directions:

Butter the crockpot well.

In a bowl, whisk the egg, coconut milk, and oil together.

Mix the dry **Ingredients**. Slowly stir in the wet **Ingredients**. Do not over mix.

Pour the batter in the crockpot, spread evenly.

Spread the berries on top.

Cover, cook on high for 2 hours. Cool in the crock for 1-2 hours.

Nutrition:

Calories: 263

Carbs: 9g

Fat: 22g

Protein: 5g

Cocoa Pudding Cake

Preparation time: 15 minutes

Cooking time: 3 hours

Servings: 10

Ingredients:

1 Tablespoon butter for greasing the crockpot

1 ½ cups ground almonds

¾ cup sweetener, Swerve (or a suitable substitute)

¾ cup cocoa powder

¼ cup whey protein

2 teaspoons baking powder

¼ teaspoon salt

4 large eggs

½ cup butter, melted

¾ cup full-fat cream

1 teaspoon vanilla extract

Directions:

Butter the crockpot thoroughly.

Whisk the dry fixing in a bowl.

Stir in the melted butter, eggs, cream, and vanilla. Mix well.

Pour the batter into the crockpot and spread evenly.

Cook within 2½ to 3 hours, low. If preferred – more like pudding, cook cake shorter; more dry cake, cook longer.

Cool in the crockpot for 30 minutes. Cut and serve.

Nutrition:

Calories: 250

Carbs: 29g

Fat: 5g

Protein: 22g

Keto Coconut Hot Chocolate

Preparation time: 15 minutes

Cooking time: 4 hours

Servings: 8

Ingredients:

5 cups full-fat coconut milk

2 cups heavy cream

1 tsp vanilla extract

1/3 cup cocoa powder

3 ounces dark chocolate, roughly chopped

½ tsp cinnamon

Few drops of stevia to taste

Directions:

Add the coconut milk, cream, vanilla extract, cocoa powder, chocolate, cinnamon, and stevia to the crockpot and stir to combine.

Cook for 4 hours, high, whisking every 45 minutes.

Taste the hot chocolate and if you prefer more sweetness, add a few more drops of stevia.

Nutrition:

Calories: 135 Carbs: 5g

Fat: 11g

Protein: 5g

Ambrosia

Preparation time: 15 minutes

Cooking time: 3 hours

Servings: 10

Ingredients:

1 cup unsweetened shredded coconut

¾ cup slivered almonds

3 ounces dark chocolate (high cocoa percentage), roughly chopped

1/3 cup pumpkin seeds

2 ounces salted butter

1 tsp cinnamon

2 cups heavy cream

2 cups full-fat Greek yogurt

1 cup fresh berries – strawberries and raspberries are best

Directions:

Place the shredded coconut, slivered almonds, dark chocolate, pumpkin seeds, butter, and cinnamon into the crockpot.

Cook for 3 hours, high, stirring every 45 minutes to combine the chocolate and butter as it melts.

Remove the mixture from the crockpot, place in a bowl, and leave to cool.

In a large bowl, whip the cream until softly whipped.

Stir the yogurt through the cream.

Slice the strawberries into pieces, then put it to the cream mixture, along with the other berries you are using, fold through.

Sprinkle the cooled coconut mixture over the cream mixture.

Nutrition:

Calories: 57

Carbs: 11g

Fat: 1g

Protein: 1g

Dark Chocolate and Peppermint Pots

Preparation time: 15 minutes

Cooking time: 2 hours

Servings: 6

Ingredients:

2 ½ cups heavy cream

3 ounces dark chocolate, melted in the microwave

4 egg yolks, lightly beaten with a fork

Few drops of stevia

Few drops of peppermint essence to taste

Directions:

Mix the beaten egg yolks, cream, stevia, melted chocolate, and peppermint essence in a medium-sized bowl.

Prepare the pots by greasing 6 ramekins with butter.

Pour the chocolate mixture into the pots evenly.

Put the pots inside the slow cooker and put hot water below halfway up.

Cook for 2 hours, high. Take the pots out of the slow cooker and leave to cool and set.

Serve with a fresh mint leaf and whipped cream.

Nutrition:

Calories: 125

Carbs: 15g

Fat: 6g

Protein: 1g

Creamy Vanilla Custard

Preparation time: 15 minutes

Cooking time: 3 hours

Servings: 8

Ingredients:

3 cups full-fat cream

4 egg yolks, lightly beaten

2 tsp vanilla extract

Few drops of stevia

Directions:

Mix the cream, egg yolks, vanilla extract, and stevia in a medium-sized bowl.

Pour the mixture into a heat-proof dish. Place the dish into the slow cooker.

Put hot water into the pot, around the dish, halfway up. Set the temperature to high.

Cook for 3 hours. Serve hot or cold!

Nutrition:

Calories: 206

Carbs: 30g

Fat: 7g

Protein: 6g

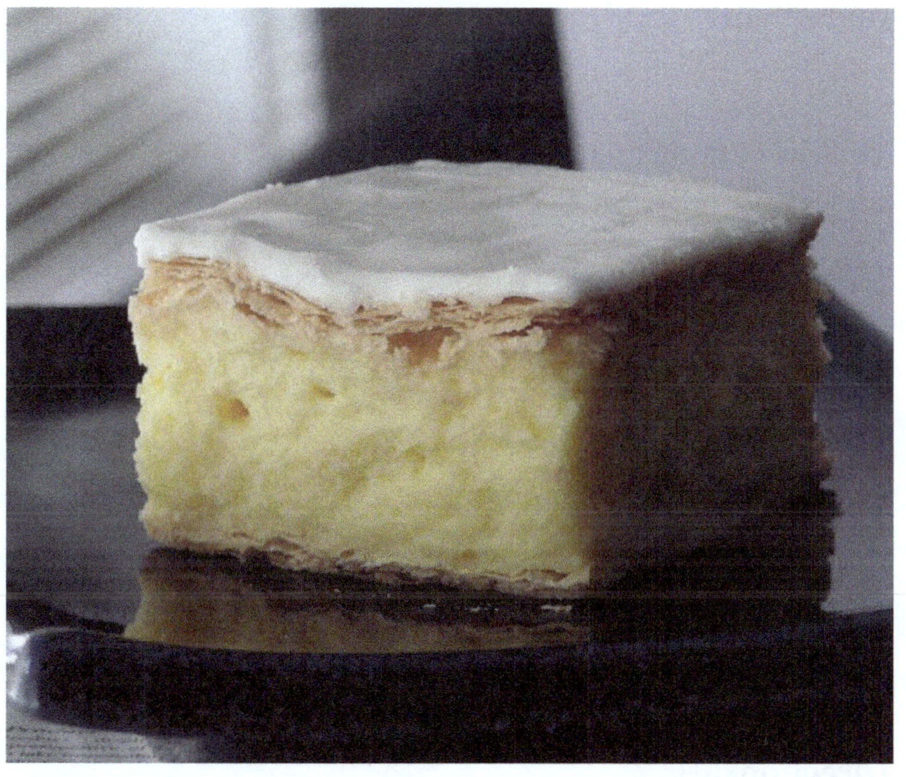

Coconut, Chocolate, And Almond Truffle Bake

Preparation time: 15 minutes

Cooking time: 4 hours

Servings: 8

Ingredients:

3 ounces butter, melted

3 ounces dark chocolate, melted

1 cup ground almonds

1 cup desiccated coconut

3 tbsp unsweetened cocoa powder

2 tsp vanilla extract

1 cup heavy cream

A few extra squares of dark chocolate, grated

¼ cup toasted almonds, chopped

Directions:

In a large bowl, mix the melted butter, chocolate, ground almonds, coconut, cocoa powder, and vanilla extract.

Roll the mixture into balls. Grease a heat-proof dish.

Place the balls into the dish—Cook for 4 hours, low setting.

Leave the truffle dish to cool until warm. Mix the cream until soft peak.

Spread the cream over the truffle dish and sprinkle the grated chocolate and chopped toasted almonds over the top. Serve immediately!

Nutrition:

Calories: 115

Carbs: 8g

Fat: 10g

Protein: 2g

Peanut Butter, Chocolate, And Pecan Cupcakes

Preparation time: 15 minutes

Cooking time: 4 hours

Servings: 14

Ingredients:

14 paper cupcake cases

1 cup smooth peanut butter

2 ounces butter

2 tsp vanilla extract

5 ounces dark chocolate

2 tbsp coconut oil

2 eggs, lightly beaten

1 cup ground almond s

1 tsp baking powder

1 tsp cinnamon

10 pecan nuts, toasted and finely chopped

Directions:

Dissolve the dark chocolate plus coconut oil in the microwave, stir to combine, and set aside.

Place the peanut butter and butter into a medium-sized bowl, microwave for 30 seconds at a time until the butter has just melted.

Mix the peanut butter plus butter until combined and smooth.

Stir the vanilla extract into the peanut butter mixture.

Mix the ground almonds, eggs, baking powder, and cinnamon in a small bowl.

Pour the melted chocolate and coconut oil evenly into the 14 paper cases.

Spoon half of the almond/egg mixture evenly into the cases, on top of the chocolate and press down slightly.

Spoon the peanut butter mixture into the cases, on top of the almond/egg mixture.

Spoon the remaining almond/egg mixture into the cases.

Put the pecans on top of each cupcake.

Put the filled cases into the slow cooker—Cook for 4 hours, high setting.

Nutrition:

Calories: 145 Carbs: 20g

Fat: 3g Protein: 4g

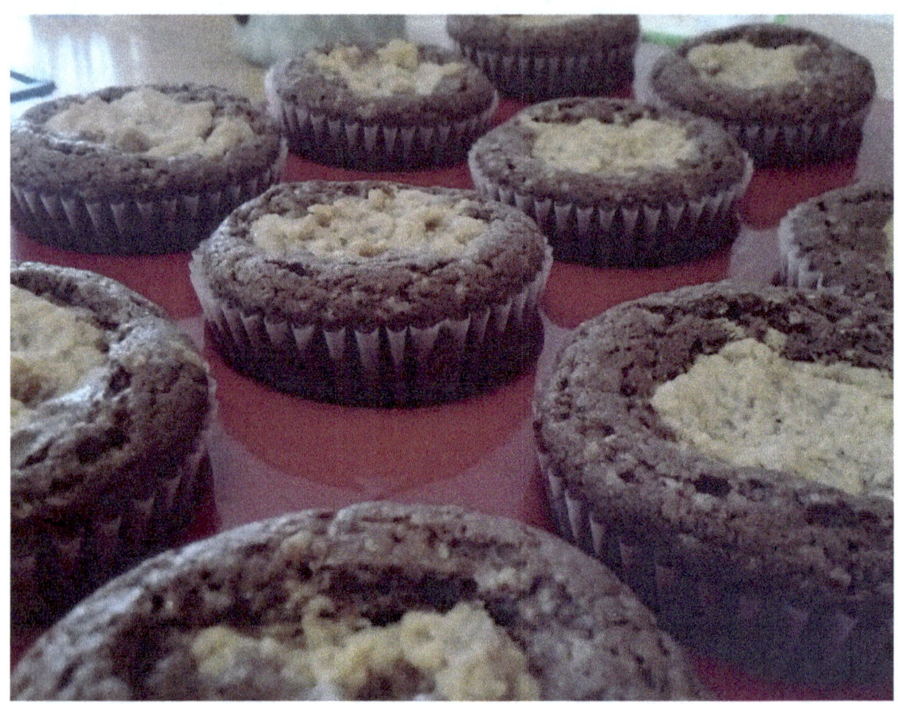

Vanilla and Strawberry Cheesecake

Preparation time: 15 minutes

Cooking time: 6 hours

Servings: 8

Ingredients:

Base:

2 ounces butter, melted

1 cup ground hazelnuts

½ cup desiccated coconut

2 tsp vanilla extract

1 tsp cinnamon

Filling:

2 cups cream cheese

2 eggs, lightly beaten

1 cup sour cream

2 tsp vanilla extract

8 large strawberries, chopped

Directions:

Mix the melted butter, hazelnuts, coconut, vanilla, and cinnamon in a medium-sized bowl.

Press the base into a greased heat-proof dish.

Mix the cream cheese, eggs, sour cream, and vanilla extract, beat with electric egg beaters in a large bowl until thick and combined.

Fold the strawberries through the cream cheese mixture.

Put the cream cheese batter into the dish, on top of the base, spread out until smooth.

Put it in the slow cooker and put hot water around the dish until halfway up.

Cook for 6 hours, low setting until just set but slightly wobbly.

Chill before serving.

Nutrition:

Calories: 156

Carbs: 4g

Fat: 7g

Protein: 15g

Coffee Creams with Toasted Seed Crumble Topping

Preparation time: 15 minutes

Cooking time: 4 hours

Servings: 6

Ingredients:

2 cups heavy cream

3 egg yolks, lightly beaten

1 tsp vanilla extract

3 tbsp strong espresso coffee (or 3tsp instant coffee dissolved in 3tbsp boiling water)

½ cup mixed seeds – sesame seeds, pumpkin seeds, chia seeds, sunflower seeds,

1 tsp cinnamon

1 tbsp coconut oil

Directions:

Heat-up the coconut oil in a small frypan until melted.

Add the mixed seeds, cinnamon, and a pinch of salt, toss in the oil and heat until toasted and golden, place into a small bowl and set aside.

Mix the cream, egg yolks, vanilla, and coffee in a medium-sized bowl.

Pour the cream/coffee mixture into the ramekins.

Place the ramekins into the slow cooker. Put hot water inside until halfway.

Cook on low setting for 4 hours.

Remove, then leave to cool slightly on the bench.

Sprinkle the seed mixture over the top of each custard before serving.

Nutrition:

Calories: 35

Carbs: 4g

Fat: 2g

Protein: 1g

Lemon Cheesecake

Preparation time: 15 minutes

Cooking time: 6 hours

Servings: 10

Ingredients:

2 ounces butter, melted

1 cup pecans, finely ground in the food processor

1 tsp cinnamon

2 cups cream cheese

1 cup sour cream

2 eggs, lightly beaten

1 lemon

Few drops of stevia

1 cup heavy cream

Directions:

Mix the melted butter, ground pecans, and cinnamon until it forms a wet, sand-like texture.

Press the butter/pecan mixture into a greased, heat-proof dish and set aside.

Place the cream cheese, eggs, sour cream, stevia, zest, and juice of one lemon into a large bowl, beat with electric egg beaters until combined and smooth.

Put the cream cheese batter into the dish, on top of the base.

Place the dish inside the slow cooker, then put warm water in halfway up.

Cook within 6 hours, low setting.

Set the cheesecake on the bench to cool and set.

Whip the cream until soft peak, and spread over the cheesecake before serving.

Nutrition:

Calories: 271

Carbs: 33g

Fat: 15g

Protein: 2g

Macadamia Fudge Truffles

Preparation time: 15 minutes

Cooking time: 4 hours

Servings: 25

Ingredients:

1 cup roasted macadamia nuts, finely chopped

½ cup ground almonds

2 ounces butter, melted

5 ounces dark chocolate, melted

1 tsp vanilla extract

1 egg, lightly beaten

Directions:

Place the macadamia nuts, almonds, melted butter, melted chocolate, vanilla, and egg into a large bowl, stir until combined.

Grease the bottom of the crockpot by rubbing with butter. Place the mixture into the crockpot and press down.

Set to cook low setting within 4 hours.

Allow the batter to cool until just warm. Take a teaspoon, scoop the mixture out, and roll into balls.

Refrigerate to harden slightly. Store the truffle balls in the fridge.

Nutrition:

Calories: 150

Carbs: 19g

Fat: 6g

Protein: 6g

Chocolate Covered Bacon Cupcakes

Preparation time: 15 minutes

Cooking time: 3 hours

Servings: 10

Ingredients:

10 paper cupcake cases

5 slices streaky bacon, cut into small pieces, fried in a pan until crispy

5 ounces dark chocolate, melted

1 cup ground hazelnuts

1 tsp baking powder

2 eggs, lightly beaten

½ cup full-fat Greek yogurt

1 tsp vanilla extract

Directions:

Mix the fried bacon pieces and melted chocolate in a bowl, set aside.

Mix the ground hazelnuts, baking powder, eggs, yogurt, vanilla, and a pinch of salt in a medium-sized bowl.

Spoon the hazelnut mixture into the cupcake cases.

Spoon the chocolate and bacon mixture on top of the hazelnut mixture.

Place the cupcake cases into the crockpot. Cook for 3 hours, high setting.

Remove the cupcakes from the pot and leave to cool on the bench before storing serving. Serve with whipped cream!

Nutrition:

Calories: 185 Carbs: 27g

Fat: 8g

Protein: 4g

Chocolate, Berry, And Macadamia Layered Jar

Preparation time: 15 minutes

Cooking time: 6 hours

Servings: 6

Ingredients:

5 ounces dark chocolate, melted

½ cup mixed berries, (fresh) – any berries you like

3/4 cup toasted macadamia nuts, chopped

7 ounces cream cheese

½ cup heavy cream

1 tsp vanilla extract

Directions:

Whisk the cream cheese, cream, and vanilla extract in a medium-sized bowl.

Scoop a small amount of melted chocolate, put it into each jar or ramekin.

Place a few berries on top of the chocolate.

Sprinkle some toasted macadamias onto the berries. Scoop the cream cheese mixture into the ramekin.

Place another layer of chocolate, berries, and macadamia nuts on top of the cream cheese mixture.

Put the jars inside the slow cooker and put the hot water until it reaches halfway up.

Set to low, then cook for 6 hours.

Remove the jars and leave them to cool and set on the bench for about 2 hours before serving.

Nutrition:

Calories: 150 Carbs: 25g Fat: 15g Protein: 3g

Salty-Sweet Almond Butter and Chocolate Sauce

Preparation time: 15 minutes

Cooking time: 4 hours

Servings: 1

Ingredients:

1 cup almond butter

2 ounces salted butter

1-ounce dark chocolat e

½ tsp sea salt

Few drops of stevia

Directions:

Place the almond butter, butter, dark chocolate, sea salt, and stevia to the crockpot.

Cook for 4 hours, high, stirring every 30 minutes to combine the butter and chocolate as they melt. Serve or store in a fridge.

Nutrition:

Calories: 200 Carbs: 21g Fat: 7g

Protein: 15g

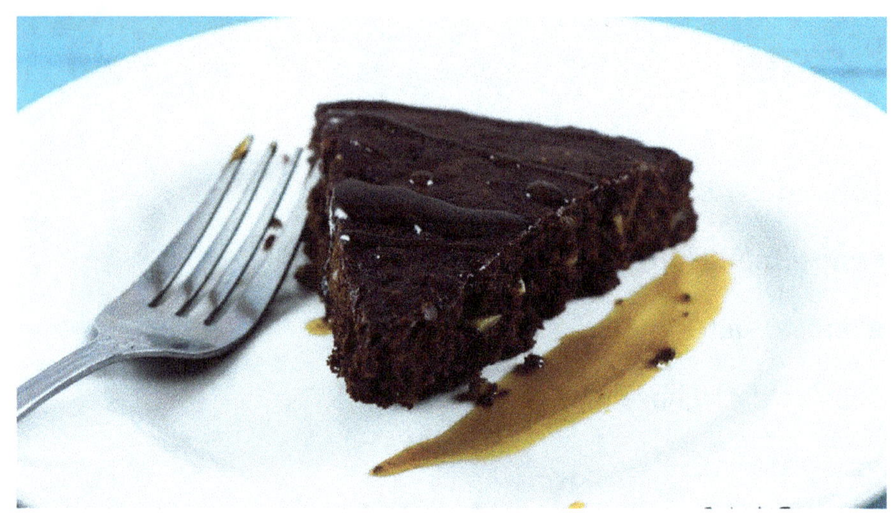

Coconut Squares with Blueberry Glaze

Preparation time: 15 minutes

Cooking time: 3 hours

Servings: 20

Ingredients:

2 cups desiccated coconut

1-ounce butter, melted

3 ounces cream cheese

1 egg, lightly beaten

½ tsp baking powder

2 tsp vanilla extract

1 cup of frozen berries

Directions:

Beat the coconut, butter, cream cheese, egg, baking powder, and vanilla extract, using a wooden spoon in a bowl until combined and smooth.

Grease a heat-proof dish with butter. Spread the coconut mixture into the dish.

Defrost the blueberries in the microwave until they resemble a thick sauce. Spread the blueberries over the coconut mixture.

Put the dish into the slow cooker, then put hot water until it reaches halfway up the dish.

Cook for 3 hours, high. Remove the dish from the pot and leave to cool on the bench before slicing into small squares.

Nutrition:

Calories: 115

Carbs: 20g

Fat: 3g

Protein: 3g

Chocolate and Blackberry Cheesecake Sauce

Preparation time: 15 minutes

Cooking time: 6 hours

Servings: 1

Ingredients:

¾ lb. cream cheese

½ cup heavy cream

1 ½ ounces butter

3 ounces dark chocolate

½ cup fresh blackberries, chopped

1 tsp vanilla extract

Few drops of stevia

Directions:

Place the cream cheese, cream, butter, dark chocolate, blackberries, vanilla, and stevia into the slow cooker.

Place the lid onto the pot and set the temperature to low.

Cook for 6 hours, stirring every 30 minutes to combine the butter and chocolate as it melts. Serve, or store in a fridge.

Nutrition:

Calories: 200

Carbs: 18g

Fat: 13g

Protein: 3g

Hot Fudge Cake

Preparation time: 25 minutes

Cooking time: 3 hours

Servings: 10

Ingredients:

1¼ cup Sukrin Gold, divided

1 cup almond flour

¼ cup plus 3 Tbsp. unsweetened cocoa powder, divided

2 tsp baking powder

½ tsp. salt

½ cup heavy cream

2 Tbsp melted butter

½ tsp. vanilla extract

1¾ cups boiling water

Directions:

Mix ¾ cup Sukrin Gold, almond flour, cocoa, baking powder, and salt. Stir in heavy cream, butter, and vanilla. Put it inside the slow cooker.

Mix ½ cup Sukrin Gold and ¼ cup cocoa, then sprinkle over the mixture in the slow cooker. Pour in boiling water. Do not stir.

Cook 2–3 hours, high. Serve.

Nutrition:

Calories 252

Fat 13 g

Sodium 177 mg

Carbs 28 g

Sugar 25 g

Protein 3 g

Fudgy Secret Brownies

Preparation time: 10 minutes

Cooking time: 2 hours

Servings: 8

Ingredients:

4 oz. unsweetened chocolate

¾ cup of coconut oil

¾ cup frozen diced okra, partially thawed

3 large eggs

36 stevia packets

1 teaspoon pure vanilla extract

¼ tsp. mineral salt

¾ cup coconut flour

½–¾ cup coarsely chopped walnuts or pecans, optional

Directions:

Melt chocolate and coconut oil in a small saucepan. Put okra and eggs in a blender. Blend until smooth.

Measure all other **Ingredients** in the mixing bowl.

Pour melted chocolate and okra over the dry **Ingredients** and stir with a fork just until mixed .

Pour into the greased slow cooker—cover and cook on high for 1½–2 hours.

Nutrition:

Calories 421

Fat 38 g

Sodium 113 mg

Carbs 15 g

Sugar 1 g

Protein 8 g

Black and Blue Cobbler

Preparation time: 20 minutes

Cooking time: 2 hours

Servings: 6

Ingredients:

1 cup almond flour

36 packets stevia, divided

1 tsp baking powder

¼ tsp salt

¼ tsp ground cinnamon

¼ tsp ground nutmeg

2 eggs, beaten

2 Tbsp. whole milk

2 Tbsp. coconut oil, melted

2 cups fresh or frozen blueberries

2 cups fresh or frozen blackberries

¾ cup of water

1 tsp. grated orange peel

Directions:

Combine almond flour, 18 packets stevia, baking powder, salt, cinnamon, and nutmeg.

Combine eggs, milk, and oil. Stir into dry fixing. Put it inside the greased slow cooker.

Mix the berries, water, orange peel, and remaining 18 packets stevia in a saucepan. Bring to boil. Remove from heat and pour over batter. Cook on 2–2½ hours, high. Let it cool within 30 minutes. Serve.

Nutrition:

Calories 224

Fat 16 g

Sodium 174 mg

Carbs 21 g

Sugar 8 g

Protein 7 g

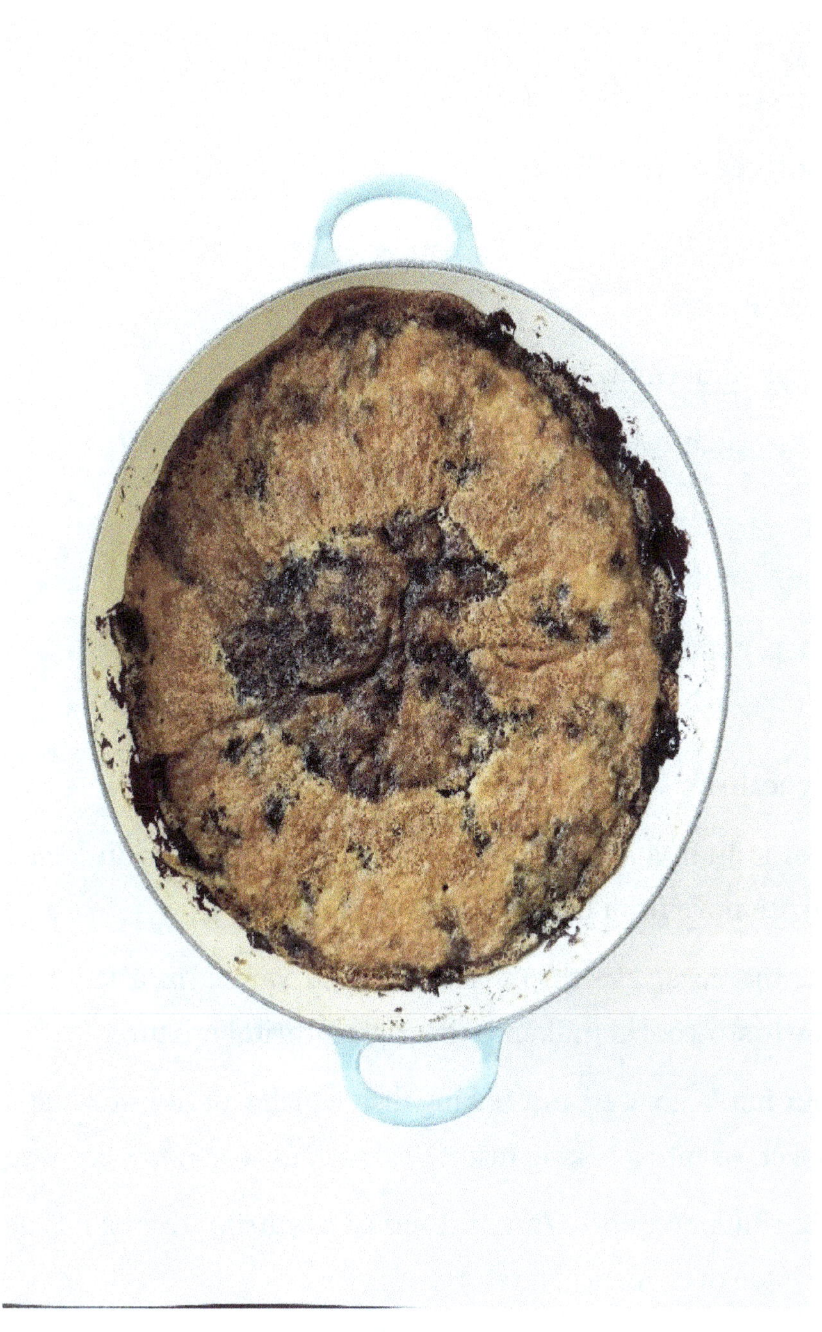

Baked Custard

Preparation time: 15 minutes

Cooking time: 3 hours

Servings: 6

Ingredients:

2 cups whole milk

3 eggs, slightly beaten

2½ Tsp., plus ¼ tsp., erythritol, divided

1 tsp. vanilla extract

¼ tsp. cinnamon

Directions:

Heat milk in a small uncovered saucepan until a skin forms on top. Remove from heat and let cool slightly.

Mix the eggs, 2½ tbsp erythritol, and vanilla in a large bowl. Slowly stir cooled milk into the egg-erythritol mixture.

Pour into a greased 1-qt baking dish which will fit into your slow cooker, or into a baking insert designed for your slow cooker.

Mix cinnamon and 1/2 tsp reserved erythritol in a small bowl. Sprinkle over custard mixture.

Cover baking dish or insert with foil—set the container on a metal rack or trivet in the slow cooker. Pour warm water around the dish to a depth of 1 inch.

Cover cooker. Cook on High 2–3 hours, or until custard is set. Serve warm from baking dish or insert.

Nutrition:

Calories 254

Fat 3 g

Sodium 6 g

Carbs 52 g

Sugar 11 g

Protein 4 g

Maple Pot de Crème

Preparation time: 15 minutes

Cooking time: 3 hours

Servings: 6

Ingredients:

2 egg yolks

2 eggs

1 cup heavy cream

½ cup whole milk

½ cup plus 1 Tbsp. Sukrin Gold

Pinch salt

1 tsp. vanilla extract

¼ tsp. ground nutmeg

Whipped cream, for garnish, optional

Directions:

Whisk the egg yolks plus eggs in al bowl until light and frothy.

Add cream, milk, 1 tbsp Sukrin Gold, salt, vanilla, and nutmeg. Mix well.

Pour mixture in a baking dish and set it in a slow cooker. Carefully pour water around the baking dish until the water comes halfway up the sides.

Cover cooker. Cook on high for 2–3 hours, until Pot de Crème is set but still a little bit jiggly in the middle.

Wearing oven mitts to protect your knuckles, carefully remove the hot dish from the cooker. Set on a wire rack to cool to room temperature.

Chill within 2 hours before you serve. Garnish with whipped cream if you wish.

Nutrition:

Calories 102

Fat 18 g Sodium 46 g

Carbs 12 g

Sugar 2 g

Protein 5 g

Slow-Cooker Pumpkin Pie Pudding

Preparation time: 7 minutes

Cooking time: 7 hours

Servings: 6

Ingredients:

15-oz. can solid pack pumpkin

12-oz. can evaporate milk

¼ cup plus 2 Tbsp. erythrito l

½ cup keto-friendly baking mix

2 eggs, beaten

2 Tbsp. melted butter

1 Tbsp. pumpkin pie spice

2 tsp. vanilla extract

Directions:

Mix all **Ingredients**. Pour into the greased slow cooker.

Cook within 6–7 hours, high. Serve.

Nutrition:

Calories 168

Fat 15 g

Sodium 91 g

Carbs 22 g

Sugar 3 g

Protein 9 g

Choco-peanut Cake

Preparation time: 15 minutes

Cooking time: 2 hours

Servings: 10

Ingredients:

15.25 oz. devil's food cake mix

1 cup of water

1/2 cup salted butter, melted

3 eggs

8 oz. pkg. mini Reese's peanut butter cups

For the topping

1 cup creamy peanut butter

3 Tbsp. powdered sugar

Ten bite-size Reese's peanut butter cups

Directions:

Mix the cake mixture, ice, butter, and eggs in a large bowl until smooth. Some lumps are all right, that's all right. Cut the cups of the mini peanut butter.

Cleaner non-stick spray on the slow cooker. Add the butter slowly and spread over an even layer.

Cover and cook on high during the **Cooking time** for 2 hours without opening the lid.

Melt the peanut butter over medium heat in a pan. Stir until melted and smooth; observe as it burns hard. To smooth, add the powdered sugar and whisk.

Pour over the butter of the sweetened peanut in the cake, then serve.

Nutrition:

Calories: 607

Carbohydrates: 57g

Protein: 13g

Fat: 39g

Saturated Fat: 13g

Crockpot Apple Pudding Cake

Preparation time: 15 minutes

Cooking time: 3 hours

Servings: 10

Ingredients:

2 cups all-purpose flour

2/3 plus 1/4 cup sugar, divided

3 tsp baking powder

1 tsp salt

1/2 cup butter cold

1 cup milk

4 apples, diced

1 1& /2 cups orange juice

1/2 cup honey

2 tbsp butter melted

1 tsp cinnamon

Directions:

Mix the flour, 2/3 cup sugar, baking powder, and salt. Slice the butter until you have coarse crumbs in the mixture.

Remove the milk from the crumbs until moistened.

Grease a 4 or 5 qt crockpot's bottom and sides. Spoon the batter into the crockpot's bottom and spread evenly. Place the diced apples evenly over the mixture.

Whisk together the orange juice, honey, butter, remaining sugar, and cinnamon in a medium-sized pan. Garnish the apples.

Place the crockpot opening with a clean kitchen towel, place the lid on, it prevents condensation from reaching the crockpot from the cover.

Place the crockpot on top and cook until apples are tender for 2 to 3 hours. Serve hot.

Nutrition:

Calories 405

Fat 9g

Saturated Fat 3g

Carbohydrates 79g

Fiber 2g

Sugar 63g

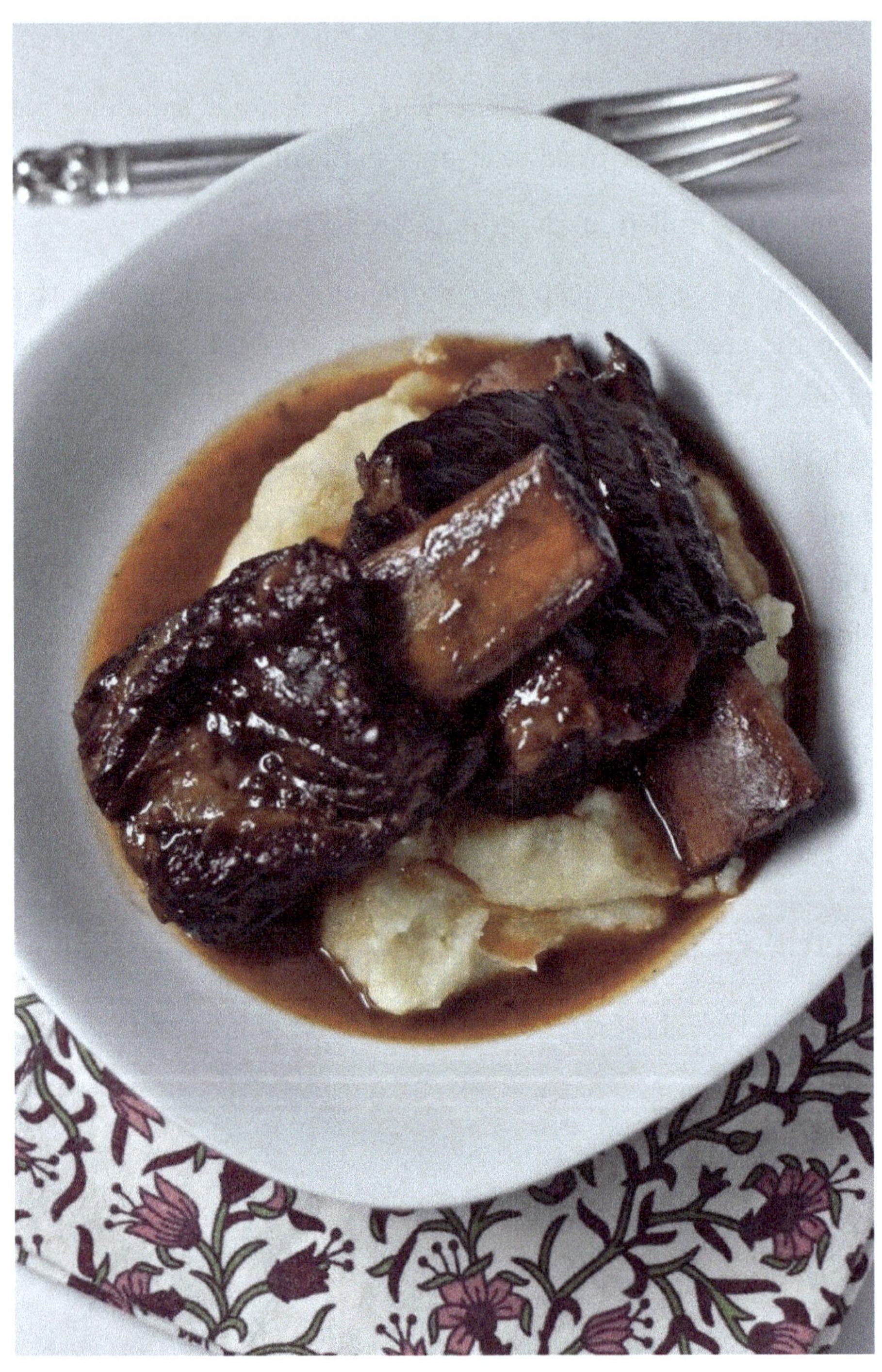

Crockpot Brownie Cookies

Preparation time: 15 minutes

Cooking time: 2 hours

Servings: 10

Ingredients:

One box brownie mix

Two eggs

1/4 c butter melted

1/2 c mini chocolate chips

1/2 c chopped walnuts optional

8 slices cookie dough slices

Directions:

Combine your brownie mixture with butter, eggs, chocolate chips, and nuts.

Sprinkle with non-stick spray the inside of your crockpot. Place eight slices of ready-made cookie dough or pile tbsp of it on the bottom.

In your slow cooker, pour brownie mixture on top and smooth out evenly. Put on the lid and cook on top for 2 hours.

To get both textures in your meal, scoop from the middle out to the edge for each serving. If desired, serve warm for best results, top with ice cream.

Nutrition:

Calories 452 Fat 21g

Saturated Fat 7g Carbohydrates 59g

Sugar 38g

Protein 5g

Crockpot Chocolate Caramel Monkey Bread

Preparation time: 15 minutes

Cooking time: 1 hour & 30 minutes

Servings: 6

Ingredients:

1/2 tbsp sugar

1/4 tsp ground cinnamon

15 oz buttermilk biscuits

20 milk chocolate-covered caramels

caramel sauce for topping (optional)

chocolate sauce for topping (optional)

Directions:

Mix sugar and cinnamon and set aside. Fill a parchment paper crockpot, cover up to the bottom.

Wrap 1 buttermilk biscuit dough around one chocolate candy to cover the candy completely, pinching the seam closed.

Place the biscuit-wrapped candy in the crockpot bottom, start in the middle of the crockpot and work your way to the sides.

Continue to wrap candy and put it in the crockpot, leaving roughly 1/2 inch between each. Repeat these steps with sweets wrapped in the second layer of biscuit.

Sprinkle the remaining cinnamon-sugar mixture on top when using all the dough and confectionery.

Cover the crockpot and cook for 1 1/2 hours on the lower side. Once cooked, remove the lid and let cool slightly.

Use the edges of the parchment paper to lift the monkey bread out of the crockpot. Allow cooling for at least 10-15 minutes.

Cut off any excess parchment paper around the edge when ready to serve. In a shallow bread or bowl, put monkey bread and drizzle with chocolate and caramel sauces.

Nutrition:

Calories: 337

Fat: 16g

Saturated Fat: 4g

Carbohydrates: 44g

Fiber: 1g

Sugar: 12g

Slow Cooker Coffee Cake

Preparation time: 15 minutes

Cooking time: 2 hours & 30 minutes

Servings: 12

Ingredients:

2 1/2 cups of all-purpose flour

1 & 1/2 cups of brown sugar

2/3 cup vegetable oil

1 1/3 cups almond milk

Two teaspoons baking powder

1/2 teaspoon baking soda

One teaspoon ground cinnamon

One teaspoon white vinegar

One teaspoon salt

Two eggs

1/2 cup chopped nuts optional

Directions:

In a large bowl, whisk in flour, brown sugar, and salt. Remove the oil until it is crumbly mixed.

In the flour mixture, combine the baking powder, baking soda, and cinnamon with a wooden spoon or spatula. In a measuring cup, place milk, oil, eggs, and vinegar and whisk until the eggs are pounded, then add to the flour mixture and stir until mixed.

Spray a non-stick cooking spray 5-7Qt slow cooker or line with a slow cooker liner. Pour into the crockpot with the batter.

Sprinkle the cake batter's nuts over the end. Put a paper towel over the crockpot insert and place the lid on top of it.

Cook within 1 hour and 30 minutes, high s or 2 hours, and 30 minutes.

Serve warm directly from the crockpot or store for up to 3 days in an airtight container.

Nutrition:

Calories: 411

Carbohydrates: 56g

Protein: 6g

Fat: 19g

Saturated Fat: 3g

Slow Cooker Apple Pear Crisp

Preparation time: 15 minutes

Cooking time: 4 hours

Servings: 8

Ingredients:

Four apples, peeled and cut into 1/2-inch slices

3 Bosc pears, peeled and cut into 1/2-inch slices

1/3 cup light brown sugar

One tablespoon all-purpose flour

One tablespoon lemon juice

1/2 teaspoon ground cinnamon

1/4 teaspoon kosher salt

Pinch of ground nutmeg

For the Topping:

3/4 cup all-purpose flour

3/4 cup old fashioned oats

1/2 cup chopped pecans

1/3 cup light brown sugar

1/2 teaspoon ground cinnamon

1/2 teaspoon kosher salt

Eight tablespoons unsalted butter, cut into cubes

Directions:

Combine flour, oats, pecans, sugar, cinnamon, and salt to make the topping. Press the butter into the dry fixing until it looks like coarse crumbs; set aside.

Coat lightly with a non-stick spray inside a 4-qt slow cooker: put apples and pears in the slow cooker. Add brown sugar, flour, juice of lemon, cinnamon, salt, and nutmeg. Sprinkle with reserved topping, gently pressing the crumbs into the butter using your fingertips.

Layer the slow cooker with a clean dishtowel. Cover and cook for 2-3 hours at low heat or 90 minutes at high temperature, remove the dishtowel and continue to cook, uncovered until the top is browned and apples are tender for about 1 hour. Serve cold.

Nutrition:

Calories: 267 Carbohydrates: 27g

Protein: 3g Fat: 17g

Saturated Fat: 7g

Fiber: 4g

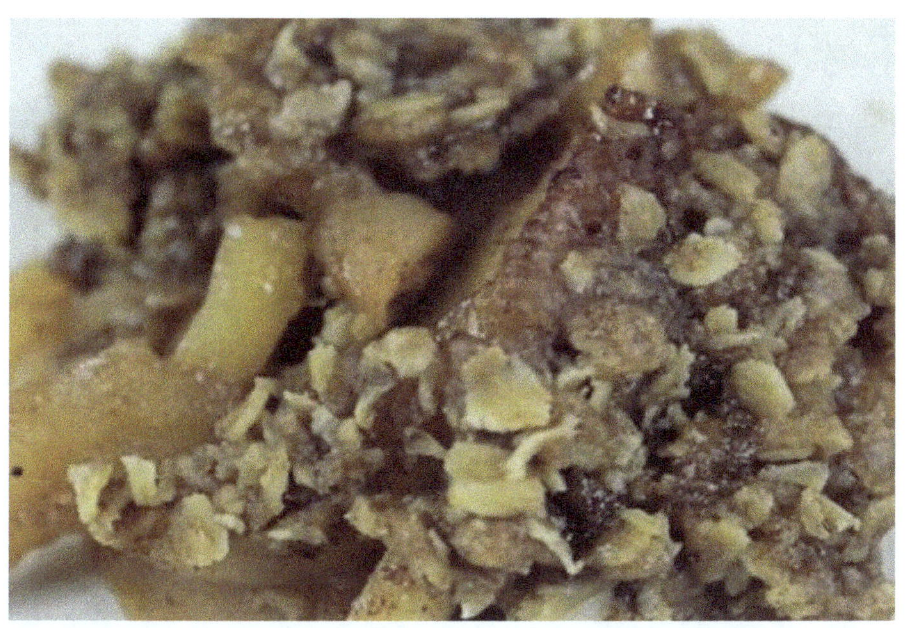

Key Lime Dump Cake Recipe

Preparation time: 15 minutes

Cooking time: 2 hours

Servings: 8

Ingredients:

15.25 oz. Betty Crocker French Vanilla Cake Mix box

44 oz. Key Lime Pie Filling

8 tbsp. or 1/2 cup butter melted

Directions:

Spray inside the Crock-Pot with a non-stick cooking spray. Empty key lime pie cans filling in the Crock-Pot bottom and then spread evenly.

Mix the dry vanilla cake mix with the dissolved butter in a bowl.

Pour the crumble cake/butter mixture over the crockpot, spread evenly, and cover the crockpot with the lid.

Cook for 2 hours at high or 4 hours at low. serve with ice cream or whip cream.

95

Nutrition:

Calories: 280 Carbohydrates: 58g

Protein: 2g Fat: 4g

Saturated Fat: 2g

Sugar: 41g

Crockpot Cherry Dump Cake Recipe

Preparation time: 15 minutes

Cooking time: 2 hours

Servings: 8

Ingredients:

15.25 oz. Betty Crocker Devil's Food Cake Mix

42 oz. Cherry Pie Filling

1/2 cup butter melted

Directions:

Spray with a non-stick cooking spray inside the crockpot.

Empty cherry pie filling cans into crockpot's bottom, then evenly spread out.

Combine dry cake mix with butter in a medium bowl.

Pour the crumble cake/butter mixture over the crockpot plus cherries, scatter

evenly, and cover the crockpot with a lid.

Cook for 2 hours at high, or 4 hours at low. Use ice cream or whip cream to serve.

Nutrition:

Calories 566 Fat 17g

Saturated Fat 11g Carbohydrates 98g

Fiber 1g Sugar 37g Protein 3g

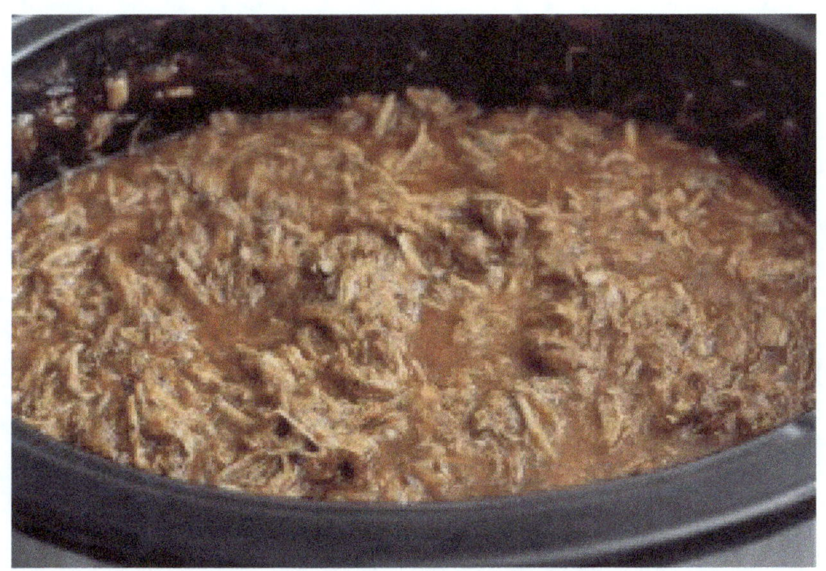

Crockpot Pumpkin Spice Cake Recipe

Preparation time: 15 minutes

Cooking time: 2 hours

Servings: 8

Ingredients:

15.25 oz. Betty Crocker Spice Cake Mix

15 oz. Libby's Pure Pumpkin

½ cup Applesauce

Three eggs

1 tsp. Pumpkin Pie Spice

Directions:

Whisk all the fixing with a mixer for 1 minute. Spray with nonstick cooking spray inside the crockpot. Pour over and cover the mixture into the crockpot.

Cook for 1.5 – 2 hours or until finished. Serve.

Nutrition:

Calories: 344 Fat: 30.38g

Carbohydrate: 10.03g Fiber: 5.61g

Protein: 8.26g

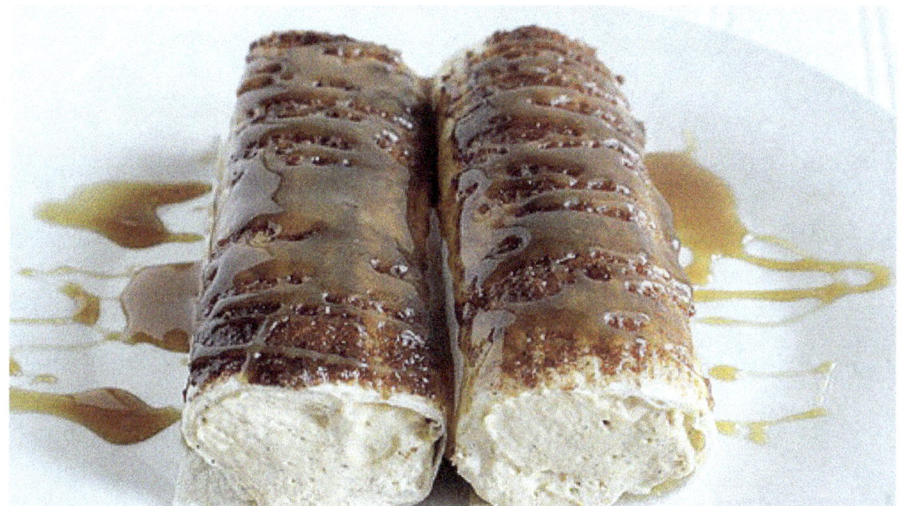

Crockpot Blueberry Dump Cake Recipe

Preparation time: 15 minutes

Cooking time: 2 hours

Servings: 8

Ingredients:

15.25 oz. Betty Crocker Lemon Cake Mix

42 oz. Blueberry Pie Filling

1/2 cup butter melted

Directions:

Spray with non-stick cooking spray the crockpot. Put blueberry pie filling evenly into the bottom of the crockpot.

In a mixing bowl, combine dry lemon cake mix with melted butter and stir until crumbly. Break some big chunks into the crumbles of a small spoon. Pour the crumble cake/butter mixture over the blueberry mixture into crockpot, spread evenly, and cover with a lid the crockpot. Cook at high for 2 hours, and at low for 4 hours. Serve.

Nutrition:

Calories: 344 Fat: 30.38g

Carbohydrate: 10.03g Fiber: 5.61g

Protein: 8.26g

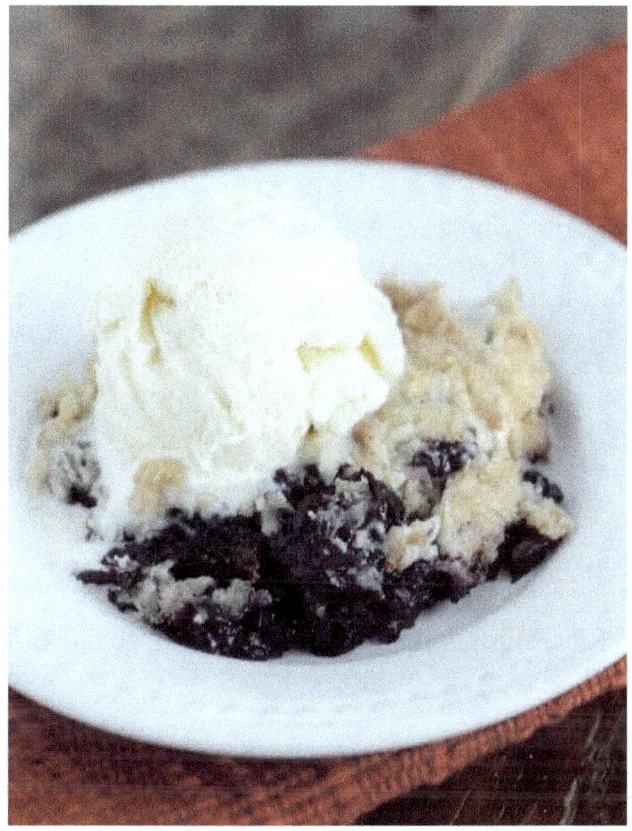

Crockpot Strawberry Dump Cake Recipe

Preparation time: 15 minutes

Cooking time: 2 hours

Servings: 8

Ingredients:

15.25 oz. Betty Crocker Strawberry Cake Mix

42 oz. Strawberry Pie Filling

1/2 cup butter melted

Directions:

Spray with a non-stick cooking spray inside the crockpot.

Put the Strawberry Pie Filling into the crockpot's bottom and spread evenly .

Combine strawberry dry cake mixture with the butter in a mixing bowl.

Pour the cake/butter crumbled mixture into crockpot over strawberries and spread evenly, covering the crockpot with a lid.

Cook for 2 hours at high, or 4 hours at low. Serve.

Nutrition:

Calories: 344

Fat: 30.38g

Carbohydrate: 10.03g

Fiber: 5.61g

Protein: 8.26g

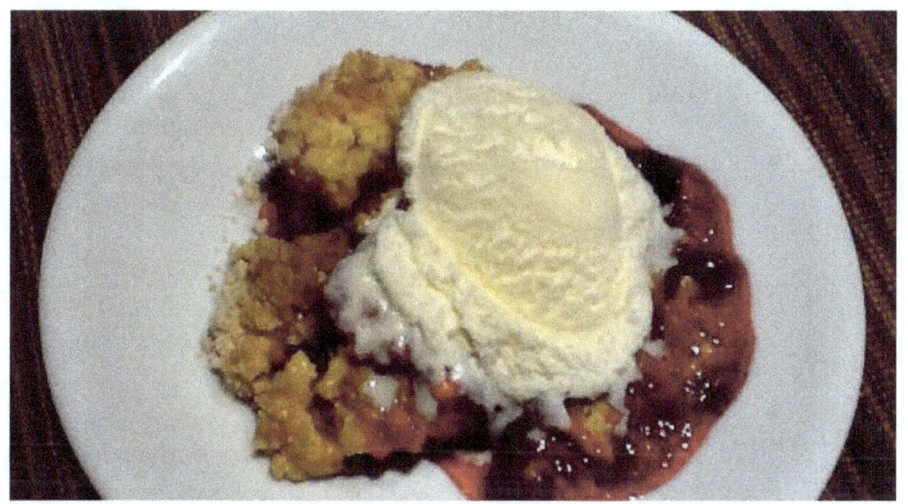

Crockpot Baked Apples Recipe

Preparation time: 15 minutes

Cooking time: 4 hours

Servings: 6

Ingredients:

Five medium Gala apples

½ cup Quaker Old Fashioned Oats

½ cup Brown Sugar

3 tsp. Cinnamon

1 tsp. Allspice

1/4 cup butter

Directions:

Pour 1/4 cup of water at crockpot's edge.

Use a sharp knife to carefully core apples.

Mix the oats, cinnamon, brown sugar, and allspice. Fill a single apple with a mixture of oats, sugar, and spice.

Use a butter pat to top each apple. Set in crockpot carefully and put the lid on crockpot.

Cook for 3–4 hours or until finished.

Nutrition:

Calories: 121

Fat 3g

Carbohydrates 48g

Fiber 5g

Sugar 36g

Protein 1g.

Sugar-Free Chocolate Molten Lava Cake

Preparation time: 15 minutes

Cooking time: 3 hours

Servings: 3

Ingredients:

1/2 cup hot water

1-ounce chocolate chips, sugar-free

1/4 teaspoon vanilla liquid stevia

1/4 teaspoon vanilla extract

1 egg yolk

1 whole egg

2 tablespoons butter melted, cooled

1/4 teaspoon baking powder

1/8 teaspoon salt

3 ¾ teaspoons cocoa powder, unsweetened

2 tablespoons almond flour

6 tablespoons Swerve sweetener divided

Directions:

Grease the slow cooker, mix the flour, baking powder, 2 tablespoons cocoa powder, almond flour, and 4 tablespoons of Swerve in a bowl.

In a separate bowl, stir in eggs with melted butter, liquid stevia, vanilla extract, egg yolks, and eggs.

Mix the wet fixing to the dry ones and combine to incorporate fully. Pour the mixture into the slow cooker.

Top the mixture with chocolate chips.

Mix the remaining swerve with cocoa powder and hot water in a separate bowl, and pour this mixture over chocolate chips.

Cook on low within 3 hours. Once done, let cool and then serve.

Nutrition:

Calories 157

Fat 13g

Carbs 10.5g

Protein 3.9g

Blueberry Lemon Custard Cake

Preparation time: 15 minutes

Cooking time: 3 hours

Servings: 3

Ingredients:

2 tablespoons fresh blueberries

1/2 cup light cream

1/8 teaspoon salt

2 tablespoons Swerve sweetener

1/4 teaspoon lemon liquid stevia

1 1/3 tablespoon lemon juice

1/2 teaspoon lemon zest

2 tablespoons coconut flour

1 ½ egg separated

Directions:

Put egg whites into a stand mixture and whip to achieve stiff peaks consistency.

Set the egg whites aside, whisk the yolks and the other **Ingredients** apart from the blueberries.

Mix the egg whites into the batter to thoroughly combine, and then grease the slow cooker.

Put the batter into it, then top with the blueberries—Cook within 3 hours, low.

Let cool when not covered for 1 hour, then keep it chilled for at least 2 hours or overnight.

Serve the cake topped with unsweetened cream if you like.

Nutrition:

Calories 140

Fat 9.2g

Carbs 7.3g

Protein 3.9g